Yoga l Beginners

Burn fat, tone up & release stress with yoga for beginners

Angela Yee

Table of Contents

Introduction

Why Should I Do Yoga?

What Is Yoga Anyway?

Top 8 Health Benefits of yoga

6 Major Types of Yoga

Basic Yoga Poses

Where To Practice Yoga

Nutrition For Yoga

Yoga Equipment & Accessories

Conclusion

Introduction

Yoga is one of the all-around most versatile form of exercise that you will find. It is designed to unite the body, mind and soul and addresses a multitude of issues that may be preventing you from getting the most out of life.

Yoga is an ancient practice, originating centuries ago in the Far East. But it has made its way the Western Civilization and is now a mainstay in the routine of many.

Whether your goal is to lose weight, tone up or to distress, Yoga has what you need. Although Yoga is much more than just meditation, it does employ meditation. Meditation will help you to reduce stress which not only calms the nerves, it also helps relieve many physical conditions like allergies, asthma, arthritis and other chronic pains.

Yoga also speeds up metabolism. That is how Yoga helps you to drop pounds. Furthermore, stress itself causes fatty build up and the slowing down of metabolism so it all works together for good.

Yoga is good for the mind and the body. They go together as a package in this form of exercise. You will gain peace of mind and serenity as well as flexibility, strength and optimal health.

This book is designed for beginners in that it gives an overall outlook to Yoga and explains the principals and practices. If you have the slightest interest in

Yoga, keep reading to find out much more about how the ancient art can help you in your everyday life.

Why Should I Do Yoga?

Yoga teaches us to cure what need not be endured and endure what cannot be cured.

-B.K.S. Iyengar

What Is Yoga Anyway?

What do you think of when you think of Yoga? If the first thing that pops into your mind when you hear the word "Yoga" is an image of people in pretzel positions on happy pills, don't worry. You are not alone.

While the practice does tend to lend itself to some interesting positions at times, the concept of Yoga is much different than you might think. While it did originate in a land far away, many years ago, it really does hit closer to home than you may realize.

Yoga is a very personalized, almost intimate, form of exercise. Think about what ails you. Are you overstressed? Do you constantly worry? Are you lacking energy? Maybe you have some physical issues that are preventing you from living life at the fullest. Picture yourself as an overcomer, having conquered your woes. THAT is the new picture of Yoga you can replace the old one with.

The quote above by B.K.S. Iyengar is much like the Serenity Prayer. It has to do with changing that which can be changed and accepting what cannot be. But how are we to know what can be changed until we explore our horizons? Yoga, in part, teaches getting past our roadblocks and exploring new possibilities. It is about going past our self-imposed limitations and reaching for more. It is personal and is spiritual and physical as well.

The word "Yoga" comes from the Sanskrit word "Yug" meaning "to join or bind, or to direct one's attention". That is exactly what Yoga is. It is, by definition, a philosophy teaching one to find and experience inner peace by controlling both the mind and body.

The earliest records indicating Yoga was practiced in a society goes back to the third century BCE and was associated with the Hindu religion. It was around 1893 when Yoga was first introduced to the West and it all happened at the World Fair in Chicago when the guru Swami Vivekananda sparked the interest of Americans and others of the Western Civilization.

In the book, *Living Yoga,* experts Georg Feuerstein and Stephan Bodian wrote about Yoga as an exercise that leads to inner and outer union, harmony and joy. "Unitive discipline" is how the sacred scriptures of Hinduism describe it. Sankrit refers to Yoga as *anada* or, the tapping into one's inner potential for happiness also termed *conscious living.*

Yogic science and philosophy delves into the belief that when a person learns to communicate with a power greater than himself (or herself), the flow with the force will enable the discovery of truth and that is when realization is birthed and with that, words, deeds and thoughts will mindful of such. In a way, it is about integrity of mind, body and soul, when one's beliefs and actions line up. It is a oneness with oneself as well as the power or powers that be.

Because Yoga is so widely misunderstood, it's important to touch on what Yoga isn't.

Yoga is NOT:

1. Calisthenics. True, there are some postures and positions that would may one think it is akin to calisthenics but those moves, such as pretzel poses and headstands, are designed to initiate communication with inner feelings rather than to achieve physical conditioning.

2. Meditation. Believe it or not, Yoga is not meditation nor is it religion. Meditation is a part of Yoga that brings one into the spiritual realm, but it is not what Yoga is all about. And likewise, Yoga is a practice within religion but…it is not what Yoga is.

All the fancy terms and philosophy aside, Yoga is a practice that just may be your ticket to a better life, both inside and out, mind and body. It is all about helping you optimize the things you can change and deal with the things you can't change. And when it's put like that…why WOULDN'T you do Yoga?

TOP 8 HEALTH BENEFITS OF YOGA

Yoga encompasses the body and the mind equally. They are one and the same in the practice of Yoga. Not that many years ago, the Western Civilization would have thought that concept to be quite odd. But there has been a new emergence in the West of realization of the correlation between mental and physical health and so that teaching lines right up with the Eastern philosophy.

Don't get me wrong, Yoga will help your body. But, it will help your mind at the same time. It helps both at the same time. There is no separation.

One reason Yoga works on the physical is that the general belief is that human beings are designed by nature to be active and agile. The belief is also that when the body is not mobile or it is unhealthy, that it is out of alignment. During a session, blocked tension and energy are released which eases or eliminates aching muscles, joints, tendons, ligaments and so on. The goal is for every part of the body to work at its maximum potential.

Perhaps the majority of people, at least Westerners, initially get involved in Yoga to improve their physical health in some form or fashion. They may want to better their good health or perhaps to rid themselves of an ailment. If that is why you have picked up this book...keep reading! You are about to learn some important ways in which Yoga can help your physical being.

The seven physical benefits of yoga that have been proven include:

1. Range of Motion and Flexibility: Stretching is a body benefit that is often overestimated. It gets your muscles and joints moving and provides oxygen to them too. It is estimated that in just 6 weeks, Yoga will increase flexibility by 35%.

2. Reduced Pain in Muscles and Joints: One reason Yoga helps relieve pain is that is encourages movement. Another reason is that it tends to elevate the mood and good feelings which help deal with pain too. In

addition, when stress is relieved, so it much of the pain.

3. Respiratory Improvement: Yoga helps to increase oxygen supply in the body. Oxygen helps to make the entire body healthy and to work at peak performance. It also helps alleviate headaches and other maladies.

4. Stronger Immunities: Practicing Yoga will help to keep your body strong and much more able to fight off diseases.

5. Higher Metabolism: Yoga helps to increase metabolism which in turns, helps you maintain a healthy weight. The body's ability to change food into energy depends on your metabolism. If you have a low metabolism, chances are good that you have weight issues. Raising your metabolism will help you burn fat and lose weight.

6. Each person has their own metabolic rate, which is affected by their lifestyle. As you become more active, your metabolic rate increases, which assists in weight loss. By focusing on different areas in the body, yoga can target the systems that are holding your metabolism back.

7. Better Sleep: When you get a good amount of quality sleep, the whole world is a brighter place. Yoga helps your body get good rest when you do sleep and also assists in providing your body with oxygen while you are asleep which is very important. Those who have sleep disorders often have to use oxygen when they sleep so they can get a good night's sleep.

8. Spinal Health: The spine plays a huge roll in how the whole body functions. Yoga helps to align the spine and also helps oxygen circulate to the pads in between the spine which in turn, helps the spine do its job better.

So as you can see, Yoga is not just about spiritual and mental improvements, it helps physically as well. Flexibility is gained over time with the postures that are practiced. That, in turn, helps lubricate ligaments, joints and tendon. Increased blood flow and oxygenation aids muscle tone and regenerates dormant muscles that have become weak due to lack of exercise. Weight loss, better sleep and lining up your spine are other benefits Yoga will bring.

Now you may be getting a glimpse as to what Yoga really is. It is balancing the mind and body to optimize both and to attain a better quality of life as a result.

In addition to medical benefits, Yoga provides other bonuses too. It increases flexibility which is important for daily activities such as walking and stair climbing. It helps you to not pull a muscle or injure yourself by falling. It helps balance as well which also helps keep you safe and free from getting injured from losing your footing. Some people are "accident prone" and tend to get hurt when doing the simplest of activities. That is often due to a lack of flexibility and/or a lack of balance. Yoga is a great solution to help those types of mishaps.

Did you know that Yoga actually massages your internal organs? It is said by some the only exercise that genuinely stimulates through your internal organs to prime them to optimal health. This stimulation helps the organs ward off disease and do their jobs in a more effective manner.

Another benefit Yoga brings to the table is that is actually detoxifies the body. By mildly and gently stretching the joints and muscles, it gives a detoxifying massage to certain organs which in turn flushing out impurities. When that happens, you will feel more energetic and full of life.

Yoga also adds muscle tone. Your body will look and feel better when you practice Yoga. With Yoga, there is everything to gain and nothing to lose (except perhaps a few pounds). So, let's get on with learning even more about the practice.

6 Major Types of Yoga

There are a number of Yoga variations. Through the years, the practice has been adapted to individual needs, beliefs, ideas and concepts. The diversity is definitely an advantage. You may find yourself drawn to one and not another or discover that one fits your needs more than the next. Let's take a look at the most popular forms of the ancient art.

THE SIX MOST POPULAR TYPES OF YOGA

1. Hatha Yoga
2. Karma Yoga
3. Raja Yoga
4. Bhakti Yoga
5. Tantra Yoga
6. Jnana Yoga

HATHA YOGA

The most commonly practiced form of Yoga in the West is Hatha Yoga. It is done so mostly for health and vitality. Stretching is a large part of this style of Yoga and is for the purpose of freeing the body up to live a vibrant, long and healthy life.

In Hatha, as in all forms of Yoga, the objective is to unite the human spirit with the spirit of the universe. Mental concentration and techniques of breathing along with stretching are used to reach the goal. When practiced properly, Hatha should provide peace and an ability to see yourself as one with the environment and the world around you.

While all variations of Yoga have things in common, the main intention of Hatha Yoga is to prepare the body in a fashion that will enable it to be enlightened and to absorb what is in store for it. When that is attained, the stress and pain will melt away, physically and mentally as well.

Hatha is found in other forms of Yoga too. Iyengar and Ashtanga involve doing Hatha. You will find it in is used in many variations of Yoga because it is so powerful.

Hatha is the perfect form of Yoga for those who have complications like spiritual or physical weakness because it will help you work on those areas. It actually encourages the body to move and to go forward to progress to a level in which the spirit will respond as well. It is important that both work together, the spirit and the physical.

Although the word Hatha is actually derived from the word "forceful", it is perhaps most endeared for its gentleness. It is a way to ease into Yoga. The two main focuses are meditation and the renewal of the body's energies to bring about optimal health.

RAJA YOGA

Raja Yoga is close in similarity to classical Yoga. It is regarded as the "royal path" because the goal of Raja is to unite the body and mind. It is thought by many to be one of the most difficult variations of Yoga because it focuses on mastery of the mind by direct control which isn't something that is instantly or easily attained.

For those who delight in meditation and are able to concentrate well, this form may be a good one for you. Raja has 8 limbs. They are:

1. moral discipline
2. self-restraint
3. posture
4. breath control
5. sensory inhibition
6. concentration
7. meditation
8. ecstasy

The objective of Raja Yoga is to find spiritual self-realization and to focus on intentionally and purposefully directing one's life force into a perfect balance of mind and emotions. To do so, this energy is moved up and down the spine and then on to a point located in between the eyebrows which is referred to as the "third eye".

Although this form of Yoga is not the simplest, it is extremely effective, especially for those who suffer with loads of stress. It is involved and requires concentration and meditation but once it is mastered, it is truly life changing.

KARMA YOGA

We hear a lot about karma these days. The word "karma" actually means "action". It refers to all actions that stem from an individual from the moment of birth all the way till death. It is optimally to be the path of doing the right things and taking the right actions and being selfless. It is often regarded as the act of relinquishing the ego in order to serve humanity and God.

It is from the teachings of the Bhagavad Vita that Karma Yoga got its roots. It is often referred to as the Hinduism New Testament. It is, in short, service to God by way of serving others. It involves doing away and detaching from self and knowing that good deeds arise in doing so.

BHAKTI YOGA

In this ancient form of Yoga, the objective is to rid oneself of all attachment and attraction for objects of pleasure and to transfer that affection to one and only one object which is God. It is about an eternal union and oneness with God.

It is taught in Bhakti Yoga that love has three levels of operation. Those are: material, human and spiritual. Love that is intellectual is said to be impersonal and based on the focus of objects and taking pleasure in them. But the goal is to not focus on such objects of pleasure and to refocus on God and things of the spiritual realm.

TANTRA YOGA

Tantra Yoga gets a lot of attention. It is regarded as the most Oriental form of Yoga by many. It is often associated with sexual rituals but although it is, or can be, sexual in nature, it is about far more than just sex.

The intent of Tantra Yoga is the transcending of self. One of the ways in which this is expressed is through consecrated sexuality but some Tantric practices actually say one should be celibate after a certain milestone in the Tantra lifestyle.

The real purpose of Tantra Yoga is to concentrate on the spiritual being within. It is all about enlightenment and sexuality is only one way in which this is attained and expressed.

INANA YOGA

Wisdom is the key in Inana Yoga. It is the pathway to wisdom. Jnana Yoga emphasizes "emptying out" the mind and the soul as well and ridding them of delusions so that a sense of reality is attained for the purpose of transformation and enlightenment.

Inana Yoga purposes to do away with obstacles such as ignorance in order to give way to discernment and discrimination. "Not this, not this," is the translation of the key phrase in Inana Yoga which is "Neti-neti". The meaning of the term is to remove all that stands in the way between oneself and total transformation.

No matter which Yoga form you find appealing or which suit the purpose you may want or need in a style, you are sure to benefit. Yoga, in all variations, is purposed to make an individual better and to optimize life and health.

Basic Yoga Poses

There are a number of Yoga poses. Each are ultimately designed to develop strength and flexibility but they are performed differently and their functions vary as well. Below are some common forms that are used.

STANDING POSES

One of the key Yoga poses is standing. While that may seem a bit odd, the purpose is to align the body and the feet. Of course, maintaining a good posture is another reason it is used. When you are not in a good posture, it is dangerous to stretch as you may do damage to your body. Standing poses help strengthen your legs and also help to promote elasticity in your legs and hips too.

SEATED POSES

To increase and develop flexibility in your lower back and hips, seated poses are often incorporated. In addition to helping your bak and hips, your groin, knees, ankles and spine benefit as well.

FORWARD BENDS

Forward bends allow you to stretch your lower back and hamstrings and to strengthen them at the same time. Tension melts away from your shoulders, back and neck and they become flexible as well. You will find the calmness comes as a result. Sometimes the strap or the black props are used in this exercise.

BACK BENDS

Back bends can assist in opening up the channels in your rib cage, hips and chest. They strengthen your arms too. Back bends add flexibility and elasticity to your shoulder area. In addition, back bends bring about tension relief in the front of your body up to your hips and help with the spinal area too and the spine is one of the central most important parts of your body so this is very vital to good health.

BALANCE

Balance poses are imperative in Yoga but they don't come easy for everyone. Sometimes they can be challenging. Balance aids in improving posture, elongating the spinal cord to help protect it from injuries and a myriad of other benefits.

Balance also helps you learn to focus on your goals and to learn to divert your attention to the matters before you. It requires concentration and will assist you in working on the level in which you do so. It is one of the poses that gets a lot of attention in that people will work on it more than some of the other poses. In doing so, tension, especially of the spine, tends to fall away. Balance and alignment follow as a result.

YOGA POSES FOR BEGINNERS

When you are just starting out, you will want to do some of the basic, simple poses so you don't get too sore or overwhelmed. If you do not master the poses and positions right off, don't be discouraged. It is progress not perfection. Make it fun and give yourself a break.

If you have any physical limitations, be sure to let your instructor know or if you are doing Yoga at home, check with your physician before beginning. There are modifications you may need to take and some things you may be advised not to do at all.

Basic beginner positions usually include balance poses, twisting poses and standing poses as well.

Some seated poses and forward and backward bends are incorporated into it as well. Usually the duration of the poses and positions are done at a shorter length to prevent injury and in order not to stress the body or the mind.

Poses and positions are designed to benefit the body. Be sure that you are doing them within the level you are at. If you are a beginner, master the beginner level before you move on. Your body and your mind will thank you for doing so.

Where To Practice Yoga

One great thing about Yoga is that it comes loaded with choices. Which type of Yoga to practice is only one of the decisions you will be able to make. Where to practice it is yet another.

Yoga has exploded in the past few years. There are yoga studios all around and chances are, there's one near you. Or, you may prefer to grab a DVD and practice in the privacy of your own home or even tune into a Yoga program on cable or paid television.

So the question is, whether to practice Yoga at home or in the studio. The answer lies within yourself. There are many things to take into consideration when you are making up your mind and all should be taken to heart. Here are some things can you may want to take into consideration:

Studio Practice

You may want to take Yoga in a studio setting if you are:

- Unmotivated. If you have difficulty in getting and staying motivated or are easily distracted or have trouble committing.

- Just beginning Yoga. If you feel you will have questions and concerns when starting your journey, you may want to go to a setting where there is an instructor to ask advice from.

- Impaired. If you have an injury or disability, you may find it more securing to be around others and to have an instructor who can oversee to make sure you are not injuring yourself more in the process of Yoga. Special modifications are sometimes available in studio settings.

But, there are those who flourish when practicing Yoga in their own home. Some don't have access to a nearby studio, have a schedule that does not work with organized classes or the reasons may be personal in nature. Home practice may be the best choice for those who:

Home Practice

- Do not live in the vicinity of a studio or work a shift lessons do not accommodate.

- Prefers to participate alone rather than in a group setting.

- Cannot afford the cost of lessons or do not wish to pay for lessons.

- Want to add home practice to your studio lessons.

Ultimately, you will do your core practice at one place or the other, your home or the studio. But there certainly is no harm in doing it at both places and in fact, it is actually a good idea. If you do your main lessons at the studio, you can make a spot in your home to practice in. If you do your lessons at home for the most part, you can visit a studio every once in a while to be sure you are doing poses correctly and to enjoy the company of others for a change.

Nutrition For Yoga

The diet for Yoga isn't all rice and sea weed, in fact, it's better than you may think. Simply following some pointers will guide you to a healthy Yoga diet using food you probably already eat. There are some guidelines you can follow that will help you chose a foods that will maximize the work you are doing in your Yoga plan.

According to ayruveda and Yoga, there are three basic types of food which are tamasic, rajasic and sattivic.

The least desireable food are Tamasic and are considered impure and to be avoided. Stale or fermented food are examples of Tamasic foods as are garlic, onions and vinegar.

Rajasic foods are strong and spicy. They are ones that stimulate the senses. Eggs, fish and meat are examples of rajasic foods. They are thought to produce a busy and restless mind and to overstimulate the mind and body.

Sattvic foods, on the other hand, are pure and good. It is the most beneficial and best way to eat where the

Yoga diet is concerned. These foods are easy on the digestion system and are calming to the body and mind such as grains, milk, vegetables and fruit.

Here is a list of just a few sattvic foods you may want to include in your diet: bean sprouts, black beans, adzuki beans, almonds, apples, asparagus, bananas, barley, basmati rice, beets, black-eyed peas, cherries, Chinese cabbage, cranberries, cucumbers, cauliflower, celery, dates, flax seeds, figs, lettuce, lima beans, lentils, kale, peaches, pecans, pineapple, oranges, plums, pinto beans, pumpkin, raisins, raspberries, rice, squash, sunflower seeds, sweet potatoes, strawberries, spinach, walnuts, yoghurt, yams, zucchini, watercress, whey, wild rice and watermelon.

Of course you do not have to eat only those items but incorporating as many as you can into your diet is helpful if you are wanting to ease into a Yoga diet. Sometimes when you make a drastic, strict change, it is easy to set yourself up to fail so simply working these foods into your diet is often more effective.

The foods that a Yoga diet avoids are ones that harm animals or are not desirable for a number of reasons. Meat and eggs are on the list of those not allowed in a strict Yoga diet. Also foods that are prepared or eaten in haste, that do not promote peace and calmness. Onions, garlic and fermented foods are a "no" as are canned foods, microwaved foods, processed foods, junk foods and fried foods as well.

You may want to consider fasting and cleansing your body before you start any change. That way you rid yourself of toxins and get a fresh start. But, that is not mandatory if you aren't into fasting or if, for medical reasons, you can't.

Another healthy thing to do is to add aloe Vera juice to your diet. Drink it as often as possible. You can add it to juice or even a shake if you have trouble drinking it alone. Eating slowly is another thing that is helpful. Savor the flavor and connect with the food you are taking in. And, eliminating red meat, at least within your comfort zone of doing so, will help you switch over to a Yoga diet and consuming as many raw, whole foods as you can is optimal as well.

The whole point of the Yoga diet is to feed the soul. Foods on the Yoga diet are intended to nurture the creation of prana which means life force. It is to bring vitality and health. A Yoga diet is also the avoidance of eating anything that is killed or harmed in the making of the food. It has a distinct focus on harmony with nature. When you consider the objectives of a good Yoga diet, how it strives to optimize the body and soul, it makes it easier to stick to the diet, or at least to bring it into your own diet more and more. The suggestions are with the aim of a spiritual path that is healthy and happy.

Yoga Equipment & Accessories

When embarking in Yoga, you will need to have some equipment and accessories at some point. Some can wait and some you will need right away. There are a myriad of Yoga related supplies to get you on your way to all that Yoga has to offer.

You can find a large variety of Yoga equipment and accessories in local sporting-goods stores and sometimes even at your local Walmart. Perhaps the best place to find them is online like on Amazon or Ebay. You may also luck out and come across second-hand things in local classified ads or from former Yogis.

Below are some things that you will most likely want to purchase at some point.

YOGA MATS

Yoga and Yoga mats seem to go hand in hand. You rarely see someone doing Yoga who is not sitting on a mat. There is a reason for that.

It can get quite uncomfortable sitting on the hard floor for a good while. It can actually be risky for your spine and other areas of your body too. Padding cushions a fall should you have one and minimizes any jerking of muscles and such.

Do be careful to purchase a good mat. There are some supermarket versions on the market that offer very little in the way of padding. A good one will not only have adequate padding but will provide a good grip on the floor too. It should generally measure 2 feet wide.

Mats come in a great array of colors, shapes and sizes. There are even mats for children. If you look around a bit, you are sure to find one that is perfect for you.

YOGA TOWEL

You will probably want to get yourself a Yoga towel. It's a handy thing to have along. You may need to wipe away a sweaty forehead or may need it for other reasons as well. There are skid-free ones available and also ones in fun "chakra" colors.

YOGA BAGS

Yoga bags are designed mostly to hold your Yoga mat so they are tubular or rectangular in size. You can also use them to hold your towel and other accessories. Generally, a Yoga bag has a shoulder strap so you can easily carry it. Some are made of nylon and some of other materials. You can find very inexpensive ones or get a top-of-the-line bag.

YOGA STRAPS

For doing a good amount of flexibility routines, you may want to get a Yoga strap. They assist you in holding your poses longer and will help you stretch your limbs as well.

YOGA SANDBAGS AND BOLSTERS

Yoga sandbags and bolsters are good to help you keep your body balance and offer support when you are doing your stretches, poses and positions. You can find them in a number of colors.

YOGA MEDICATION CHAIRS, CHAIRS, BENCHES, AND PILLOWS

When you are meditating or doing your Yoga exercises, there are things that are nice but not necessary to have.

One is a backjack meditation chair. It basically is a chair with no lets but offers a firm back support. There are meditation benches available in all shapes and sizes that are especially nice if there is more than one person who practices. Another nicety is the breathing, or prayanama, pillow.

YOGA BALLS

Yoga balls can be purchased for around $25 and are great to have. You can use them to help you build strength and muscle tone and balance as well. You've probably seen the standard exercise ball on which many do various types of exercises. In Yoga, the ball is used for backbends, restorative pose, hip-openers and so on. You may also want to purchase an air pump to have available for when the ball deflates.

Balls are good for building strength, achieve balance and tone muscles and can even be used as chairs to sit in while watching TV as the slight rotation you will get is good for your back and spine.

YOGA BLOCKS

Yoga Blocks are pretty common for use when practicing Yoga. They look like little padded blocks and are padded. They are fantastic for extension movements.

YOGA VIDEOS/DVDS

For times that you can't make class or if you chose to do Yoga in your home, or, if you just want to add some sessions to your normal classes, you may want to pick up a Yoga DVD. It's nice to be able to rerun certain parts until you have mastered them or be able to stop it and restart it later.

YOGA MUSIC

There are CD's that are available that will help you in your meditation. Some even assist you in perfecting your moves, breathing deeper and holding positions for a longer length of time. There are some that also aid enhance meditation and some that are designed to induce a trance-like state. Yoga audio books can also be found.

YOGA CLOTHING

You will be a lot more comfortable and will be able to perform Yoga better if you have clothing that moves along with you. While it is not mandatory, it is very helpful to have Yoga clothing. Loose-fitting t-shirts and stretchable leggings are fine for Yoga or you can find specialty work-out attire in many stores and online as well.

Be sure what you choose is comfortable so you can do your stretching and poses with ease and relaxing as well. The perfect Yoga clothes are the ones that allow for free movement and do not distract or disturb you in any way. Be sure the fabric feels good on your skin.

It's great if you find Yoga clothing that is absorbent. You may find that you perspire a bit while practicing so athletic type fabrics are great or cotton is good as well. The better you feel about your Yoga clothing and the better they feel on you, the better you will do in your sessions.

Here are a few things to watch for when you are looking for Yoga attire:

1. Yoga Tops – When practicing Yoga, you will be doing moves that could make your top fall into your face. It is important that you at least attempt to find a shirt that will not do so. Staying away from very long and lose t-shirts is advised for this reason.

2. Sports Bra- Although it is optional, you may want to purchase a sports bra to wear. When stretching, you may find you "fall out" of a

regular bra and a sports bra will help to prevent that.

3. Yoga Pants- Choosing good pants for your Yoga training is imperative. You certainly don't want to wear blue jeans or pants that restrict your movement. A good pair of leggings or stretchy-type pants are optimal. Spandex fabric is great. Attention to the length is important. You don't want your pants to be too long or you will possibly trip over them or get hung up on them when doing your poses and positions.

4. Yoga Shorts- Yoga shorts are an alternative to Yoga pants. They eliminate the possibility that you may trip over your pants. If you are comfortable wearing shorts, this may be a good option for you, especially if you are practicing Bikram Yoga which is also known as hot Yoga where the temperature is hot.

Conclusion

We as humans operate on the "pay-off system". We tend to do things based on what we get out of it. It's not a bad thing. In fact, it is a very natural process that is not limited to humans. Animals do it too.

Even things done unselfishly are done...selfishly. Not in a negative realm but because giving makes one feel good or helping someone brings a warm fuzzy feeling.

The good news is that the "pay-off system" fits right in to Yoga. In striving to unite body and mind and to live in complete harmony, there is a pay-off. Your body reaps benefits as does your mind and your spirit. Those around you will benefit as well. You will most likely live a longer and happier life when you practice Yoga.

If you are debating whether to take up Yoga or not, you might ask yourself, "What Yoga can do for me?" Chances are the pay-off will be immense and life changing!

CPSIA information can be obtained
at www.ICGtesting.com
Printed in the USA
LVOW13s1743050218
565344LV00045B/2627/P

9 781508 882084